Like Night and Day

Table of Contents

Acknowledgments

First I am eternally grateful to the Almighty God who gives me strength to accomplish all things through Christ.

I acknowledge my mother and grandmother (Tammy and Lula) who instilled so much love, wisdom and encouragement into my life. Although they are no longer with me in body, the memories I have of those two ladies are worth more than I could ever express.

I thank my sister and brothers (Tameria, Brian and Alan) for their constant love and support. I'm honored to be the eldest brother and all three of them make me so proud. I thank my nieces and nephew (Taniya, Talaya, Treniya, Tremiya and Ayden Jermaine) for giving me even more reasons to love life. I thank my extended brother and sister for their love, support and hospitality (Shon and Kim).

I thank my dad and his wife for their support and kindness (A.J. and Betty).

I would like to acknowledge and thank my primary doctor (Dr. Linda Ly - Kelsey Seybold, Houston, TX) and my surgeon (Dr. Felix Spiegel, Houston, TX) for their thorough care and masterful medical skills.

To all of my church family (1st Macedonia - Pastor Lewis, New Life in the Word - Pastor Barrett), friends and relatives - thank you for your prayers. To everyone who has connected with me and keeps me motivated and encouraged - thank you. There wouldn't be enough room for me to name everyone so please pardon my summarizations.

Lastly, I thank you for investing in me by reading this book. I pray it's a blessing to you and others and I look forward to our continued journey together.

Intro

Please Allow Me to Re-Introduce Myself

"Is that really you?" "Is this real?" "Is it photo-shopped?" "Is the guy on the left your dad?"

These are all frequently asked questions that I have the privilege to answer these days concerning my before and after pictures. I don't get offended when someone finds my journey hard to believe. I still look at my own pictures and find what I see hard to believe. Except it's not the after photo that is unbelievable to me, it's the before. WOW! Was I really that huge? Did I really walk around with well over 400 pounds of weight? The unfortunate answer is yes. I lived it, I suffered through it but most importantly I overcame it.

If you had told me just a few years ago that I would be inspiring others all over the world, jogging around my block and wearing slim-fit suits to work – I would've thought you were intoxicated. If you had told me just a few years ago that I'd have people asking me for fashion advice, complimenting my attire, calling me handsome and inquiring if I was a fashion designer or health coach - I would've thought you were insane. Well if not insane, maybe just a little too optimistic. It's hilarious to see the look of total oblivion when someone sees me who hasn't seen me in a while. They have no idea who I am until I smile and say my name. I'm told my smile has remained. My smile is connected to who I am on the inside so I'm not surprised it stayed the same. I made a deal with myself before the transformation that I would remain humble and approachable no matter what. Besides, I don't take full credit for this wonderful change. God has truly performed a miracle in my life by empowering me to make the necessary changes for a better quality of life and longevity.

"...weeping may endure for a night, but joy cometh in the morning" {Psalm 30:5}

When I think of where I was and where I am right now it's truly like night and day. I can't think of a better way to describe it. The weight loss has been a blessing, but there has been so much more to this journey than just losing excess fat. I feel as though I've been reborn. It's as if I was locked in a dark dungeon my whole life but suddenly one morning the chains were broken and a door opened revealing sunlight.

I'm a very private person by nature. People who I work with would probably describe me as nice but too quiet. I'm not very talkative and I'm certainly not used to sharing the personal details of my life with the masses. But how can I keep such an awesome testimony to myself when it could bless someone with renewed hope? God allowed me to go through this journey so that people can know that all things are possible. Yes anything bad can happen, but this is where we can get excited – ANYTHING GOOD CAN HAPPEN TOO! No matter how rough my day is, when I say that simple phrase of faith, life leaps inside of me.

I understand that it's not easy for everyone to get excited just yet. Perhaps you've been in a certain situation for so long that you've just accepted it and given up on seeking for better. Maybe you've tried and tried only to fail and fail miserably. You may not have anyone in your life to cheer you on, pray you through or hold your hand. Don't be discouraged if the people around you are not giving you the encouragement you need – even if you give it to them. It's somewhat unfair for us to expect to receive from people what they don't have to offer.

*"**We** will lift up **our** eyes unto the hills, from whence cometh **our** help. **Our** help cometh from the Lord, which made heaven and earth."* {Psalm 121:1-2}

Notice how I was inclusive when sharing that verse of encouragement. One of the hardest challenges in meeting goals and

trying to fulfil dreams is feeling alone.
Sometimes it would be nice to just have
someone to talk to who understands. If you're
anything like me you don't like burdening
people and you certainly don't want to appear
weak. I want you to know that you are not
alone. I'm right there with you. Through the
strengthening of Christ I was able to stop
dying and start living.

"Brethren, I count not myself to have apprehended:
but this one thing I do, forgetting those things
which are behind, and reaching forth unto those
things which are before…" {Philippians 3:13}

Please know that I haven't "arrived",
but I'm arriving. I still have many goals and
dreams that I'm working to fulfil. There are
principles that allowed me to go from 440
pounds to 190 pounds, from walking with

severe back pain to jogging pain-free, from sorrow to joy, and from victim to victor. These same principles can be used to help us move forward and accomplish seemingly unreachable heights.

If you or someone you know understands what it's like to struggle and seemingly have no way out, I pray that by the time you finish this book your faith will be increased. I pray that you will receive wisdom (to know how), courage (to move forward no matter what) and power (to make the challenging steps to reach whatever your goals may be). I pray that through my honesty you will realize you don't have to allow what happened before to keep you from what can happen now. You do not have to allow what someone did to you to keep you from being a blessing to others. No matter how hopeless it may seem, no matter how far away your dreams may feel – you too can have a before and after testimony. Your health, wealth, ministry, career and family can be healed, restored and catapulted to a place of thriving. Yes, I'm talking about a change like night and day.

Chapter 1
<u>Good Evening</u>

When I was super morbidly obese, people questioned why I didn't just lose weight. They wondered why I didn't just exercise or change the way I was eating to melt the excess pounds. People would offer such matter-of-fact opinions and advice that you would think I just woke up one day and decided to be super morbidly obese. When people ridicule others they often forget there are things that happen in people's lives that cause them to be in unpleasant situations. We see the *what* and fail to consider the countless *whys*. Judgmental people don't take the time to consider the root possibilities of someone's misfortune. Because I've been through so much in my life I never judge a person based on what they are dealing with. I have a firsthand understanding that there are 'whys' in everyone's life. I've learned through my own experiences and through watching others that it's best to pray, help or just stay out of other people's affairs. Any of us can be up today and down tonight. All it takes is one pregnancy and you can possibly lose your perfect figure. Just one unfortunate accident and a perfect face could need multiple reconstructions. One unfortunate incident and your sprawling home could be turned into a heap of ashes. One twist or turn in the market and a multi-million dollar business could go bankrupt. We see and hear about these kinds of stories everyday but yet some people find it hard to be empathetic concerning the misfortunes of others.

Imagine this. It gets late, the street lights are starting to show their dull glow. Mom is calling out from the kitchen window "It's time to come in". You run up to the window with hope of negotiating more play time. The smell of deliciousness from the dinner she's been working on seeps through the window screen and causes you to forget about pleading your case. Evening time may not have been the best because play time was over, but it wasn't so bad because something good was waiting inside. Evening time reminds me of my childhood because it precedes the night. There's an evening to the night season of my life.

Overall, I had a good childhood despite certain circumstantial occurrences that I'll share another time. I had a God-fearing, amazing, hard-working and nurturing mother.

I had a hard-working dad, and younger siblings that I adore. I had grandparents (especially grandmothers) who treated me like I was the last surviving prince of a sprawling kingdom. I got most of what I asked for on my Christmas lists. I went to school neat and clean, and I went to church with a heart of worship. We were not wealthy or well off – but we were fine. So why was I depressed? Part of it was because while we were fine – I was fat. Oh yes, the struggle started early. I've been obese most of my life. My siblings and I ate the same foods and played the same games outside but they were hot and I was not. They were fab and I was flab.

I can't tell if fat led to depression, or if depression just led to more fat. Maybe it was a mix of both but either way, it was a problem. I remember having these periods of paralyzing sadness that made it hard to even fake a smile. Some of the sadness was due to me feeling so alone. I've always been unique. I can remember older saints joking with each other and calling me an old man trapped in a young boy's body. I would get a good chuckle out of that and felt proud that an older generation considered me to be mature. But I wanted to be accepted by my generation too. I remember feeling so alone all of the time. Surrounded by classmates at school, surrounded by members at church, surrounded by family at gatherings – none of it mattered. I always felt like I was on an island with only me and a desire to be normal. Amongst my peers I felt chubby, not cool and unpopular.

To make social matters worse, the things I was interested in were such a contradiction to that of most young people my age. It seemed that most of the guys my age were interested in girls, gangster rap, sports, drugs, drinking, tattoos, more girls, 'ballin' (showing off) and disrespecting authority. My interests were pleasing God, family, trying to be an example for my siblings, only dating one girl at a time, success, cooking and worship themed music. I'm not at all bragging about being the perfect kid, because I wasn't. I'm just telling you how things were from my perspective. If you're assuming I spent many days eating lunch at a table alone, your assumption is totally correct.

The Big Fat Mystery

I just didn't understand why I was so overweight. Sure, I had my pig-out moments. I ate pizza, nachos, cookies, ice cream, fried chicken and ham sandwiches. Before you judge me, I wasn't the only one. Everyone I knew ate the same foods. I ate just like other growing youngsters my age. Seems that my grow-up was more like a grow-out. While my peers were getting taller, more attractive and appealing, I was getting fatter. So here it is – I'm overweight, I'm a church boy, I speak proper English and fear God. No wonder I felt like such an alien amongst the hip young people.

I saw the way girls looked at the slim athletes, or the suave pretty-boys, and "rough neck" gangsters. They looked at them like a greedy overweight kid looking at a honey-baked ham, or me looking at a honey-baked ham. I noticed the way people cleaved and catered to attractive people. I desired to be admired in that way. I actually remember sitting in class and one of the somewhat popular girls looked at me and said "if you lose weight, grow your hair out a little and get

a gold tooth, you would be kind of cute". I
don't know her name, and I can't even recall
exactly what she looked like. But I remember
those words as if they were spoken just now. I
remember going out to eat when I was a child
after church and one of the members looked at
me in the meal line and said, "You need to do
something about that weight. Women don't
want a fat man. Men are ok with fat women,
but no woman wants a fat man". Words work
as both seeds and nourishment for seeds that
are already planted. I had already planted a
seed in my own self by believing I was
unattractive and undesirable. The words from
the cool girl, and the *keepin-it-real* church
woman nourished those negative seeds and
left a stain on my memory. I should have
dismissed those words immediately as they
were spoken, but I was in agreement with
them so I allowed the words to be planted into
my thoughts. We must be careful of what

words we allow to be planted into our hearts
and minds. We must also be mindful of who
we allow to plant them. There's nothing
wrong with constructive criticism or
suggestions of improvement – but if it's not
edifying, it needs to be rejected.

I'm sure by now some are ready to
preach to me about how my worth is not
weighed by how others see me. I'm sure
someone is ready to send me a flaming note
letting me know that as long as I have King
Jesus that should be enough. I'm sure
someone wants to remind me that it's what's
on the inside that counts. I know all of this and
I do agree. But can we please stop being deep
super saints for a moment and just be real.
Sometimes I want to feel sexy. Sometimes I
want to feel desired, loved and adored by

another person – not just God. I'm just being
honest.

So there I was – depressed, unattractive,
lonely, strange (unique), unhappy and
overweight. This was my adult starter
package. Ouch!

The Cool of the Evening

Despite being overweight and under-
happy, I managed to find a wife. Before you
crack open the champagne bottles and start
throwing the confetti – the marriage was very
short lived. We divorced soon after saying I
do. Why? What happened? I won't go into
those details because the real 'why' doesn't
matter. I took full blame and responsibility for
my marriage failure. I thought I should've

been more handsome, sexier, more charming, and more successful. In my mind it ended because I was inadequate, and a total disappointment that didn't deserve a wife anyways.

Mind you, in the midst of dealing with life, I'm dieting and trying to improve my life. The diets just aren't working. I was just starving myself only to lose a few pounds and gain even more. I'm taking diet pills, staying up late watching infomercials and ordering money-wasting gimmicks in the hopes of finding a miracle cure for my fat problem. I've never been one who enjoys exercise but sometimes I would force myself to do it. Again, I'd lose a few pounds but gain even more. I told myself that it was my fault that nothing I was trying was working. I told myself that it was because I was fat and lazy and just not trying hard enough. I told myself that I couldn't stick to the strict diets because I was weak.

Just when I thought life really couldn't get much worse, it did. The lady who seemingly made my life bearable, the Olivia Pope of our family, the prayer warrior and provider – died. God saw fit to give my mother her rest at only 49 years old. I had just lost about 50 pounds right before this happened. I was so sad and depressed after losing my mother that I just didn't care to diet anymore. I ate and slept my way up to approximately 460 pounds. I say approximately because I was too heavy for my doctor's scale to get an accurate number.

So at this point I was divorced, super morbidly obese, weird (unique), tired, depressed, sad, lonely and a momma's boy with no mom. Oh, it was getting late in the evening my friends and the sun was going down.

Chapter 2

The *not-so*-Goodnight

During the evening time, there's at least a little faded sunlight to remind us of morning. Imagine a night when it gets dark and not even the bug bothered street lights can stand up to the suffocating darkness that fills the atmosphere. The birds are no longer chirping, the children are no longer playing and it's just quiet. I'm not referring to the quiet of peace and serenity. It's the quiet of emptiness and loneliness. The kind of quiet that makes you feel abandoned and rejected. The kind of quiet that leaves you with nothing to entertain yourself with but thoughts of regret and a reflection of everything you wish you could instantly change. This is how adulthood was for me.

Many chubby kids eventually grow out of it, I grew further into it. Yes, I did have times as an adult where I would lose a noticeable amount of weight. But this was due to unrealistic dieting. Once I got tired of starving myself, I would go back to eating normally and then came more pounds. I kept getting fatter. With more fat came more depression. More depression led to self-destructive thoughts. They were thoughts of unworthiness, undesirableness and even death. Now I would never commit suicide, but the thoughts were there. *I told you I would be honest with you and I'm keeping my word.*

Up until my late 20s, I was fat but ok. I could walk just fine, sleep just fine, and didn't have any serious health issues that I knew of. But soon I noticed I had to stop for a moment when walking. I noticed I was moving slower than everyone else although I almost felt like I was running a marathon. I can remember waking up in the middle of the night and I couldn't breathe. I didn't say it was hard to breathe. No, I couldn't breathe at all! My lungs were not working. I sat up in bed but that didn't help. I stumbled my way to the bathroom. I couldn't call out for help so I began to pound my chest with my fist. It worked! I started breathing again. I knew then that if I didn't resolve my health issues, I would die very soon. I didn't share this with anyone, but I predicted that I would probably live to 30 or 35. I couldn't see myself living much longer than that, and honestly didn't really want to.

You may be wondering - where were my family and friends during all of this? They were around. There was nothing they could do about any of this. I was good at keeping a façade. I was scamming those around me. Not by scamming them out of their money, but by making them believe I was ok. Why did I do that? Because I was the strong one. I was the oldest sibling who had to play third parent when my parents divorced. My mom worked three jobs at one point, so I felt obligated to be responsible for assisting her to manage the daily routines of family life. This was my doing, not hers. I've always felt this kind of obligation to everyone except myself. I always felt like I was someone that should be depended on and not felt sorry for. I needed to be someone who had it all together. In my mind, I had no right to not be ok. I didn't have a right to need counseling. I blamed myself for all of my failures so my punishment to myself was – just deal with it.

What's ironic about all of this is I'm a natural born encourager. While dealing with these thoughts and feelings of total uselessness and failures – I was ministering to people. I'd decree and declare to others that the worst was behind them and better days were ahead. I'd get hugs and encouraging feedback from people telling me how I was such a blessing. I'd get love notes from people saying that the words I spoke or shared via social media were refreshing and helpful. After the powerful me would show up and show out for others, I had to go home and deal with the pitiful me.

Long Night

I remember going out to eat with my family one night. We agreed to meet some new friends there. Unfortunately for me, the only table available was a booth. Can you imagine how embarrassed I was trying to squeeze in but couldn't? I felt like such an inconvenience to everyone. We actually had to wait additional time for a table to open up – all because I was too fat. I found the embarrassment of being super morbidly obese almost too much to bear. I began to hate to go out in public. I would make excuses when my family and friends asked me to join them. I wasn't too busy. I was just too ashamed.

I can remember another instance when my family went on a small road trip to see my youngest brother graduate from Air Force training. After the ceremony, we were all so proud of him and he was so excited to show us his new military life. The family agreed to walk to his living quarters. As the eldest brother I wanted to be ahead of the line. However, I was so exhausted and in pain from carrying around so much weight that I just couldn't make the trip. I had to go sit in the hot car and watch them walk away and fade into the distance. Here it is my baby brother, of whom I'm so proud, is trying to share his achievement and I'm too big and unhealthy to even take the stroll. It was this moment, among others, that really helped me to realize that bad health was cheating me out of life. It wasn't only cheating me, but it was cheating those closest to me who needed and wanted my support.

There was a small faint voice deep down in me saying, "I want to live and be happy". I wanted to be normal. I didn't choose to be too big to even fit into a restaurant booth. I didn't choose to be seemingly the largest person at my place of employment and church. I didn't choose to be the fattest among family and friends. I most definitely didn't choose to be so huge that I couldn't shop for clothes in normal stores. I was confined to big and tall specialty shops – and it wasn't because I was tall.

I know what some are probably thinking at this point. If I was so unhappy being fat, why didn't I just lose weight? For some it's as easy as eating a salad, doing jumping jacks and drinking water. For me, nothing seemed to work. When it did work a little, it didn't work long enough to put a substantial dent in the 250 pounds that I really needed to lose.

Chapter 3

The Breaking of Day

Don't let the upbeat tone of the title of this chapter trick you into celebrating too soon. I was still super morbidly obese at this point. My health was getting worse. I remember looking out of my window on a beautiful Saturday morning, but all I could do was lie in my bed and cry. My back was in so much pain – traumatized from trying to support 440 - 460 pounds of grown man. My legs and knees were exhausted and I was getting very close to needing a cane (in my 20s). I developed acid reflux which caused stomach acid to make its way up to my air passages and throat. This caused me to choke and feel burning pain. I had sleep apnea and was prescribed a BiPap machine to sleep with at night. The mask was very uncomfortable and I would snatch it off in my sleep. I would stop breathing so much that I would wake up feeling as though I hadn't slept at all. I began to experience shortness of breath and frequent headaches which prompted me to go to the doctor. My blood pressure was high and my EKG tests returned with abnormal results. I hadn't succumbed to heart failure yet, but I was experiencing the symptoms of it. I thought to myself, that's it! At this rate I won't live to see 30 years old.

I'm the good listener, but who could I talk to? I didn't want the people around me to know how messed up I was. I didn't want to be pathetic. I didn't want anyone feeling sorry for me. I felt so powerless against this fat problem and was getting very close to just giving up on living a happy life. I opened my bible.

"For I reckon that the sufferings of this present time are not worthy to be compared with the glory which shall be revealed in us." {Romans 8:18}

I had to have an honest conversation with God. This time I wasn't asking for the anointing to accomplish a ministry task. I wasn't asking for power from on high so that I can help pray someone else through. I came to God as His child who was in trouble. I reminded Him that although I hated life, I never stopped loving Him. I never stopped serving Him even when it was hard. I worshipped while I was weary. I was faithful while I was fat. I was dependable while I was depressed. I was helpful while I was hurting. I understand there are heavenly treasures waiting for us, but I really felt there were some heaven-on-earth treasures that I just hadn't tapped into yet. I experienced the sufferings of this present time, but I wanted to experience the glory that would become of it.

After I prayed, I had to get over myself. If we're going to depend on God to lead us to a better life we must be flexible to new methods. I had to forgive myself for failing before and be willing to accept a new day. I had to quit holding myself to unreasonable scrutiny. It's ok to need help sometimes. It's ok to admit we don't have all the answers.

At this point God knew I was ready for my daybreak. My night season was long, but it was over. He began to lead and guide me to the right professionals and specialist and people who already experienced triumph with weight loss. No more pride! I was open and receptive to do whatever it took for me to finally reach this goal of being healthy.

I researched and found a surgery that I believed would help me get rid of some weight fast so that I can start exercising. I was tired of feeling like I was four times the age I actually was. My change was past due. I definitely hit some obstacles along the way. If we wait until it's easy to make a change, we'll never get it done. There are many hurdles, ditches and rough stretches of road to overcome on our way to victory. The first surgeon I called didn't work out. He was more concerned about my money than he was my health. Seriously! Most of my initial consultation with him was all about money. I couldn't believe it! Here I am almost in the grasp of death at an early age, about to allow someone to change my internal anatomy and this man is talking to me about money. Of course I knew it wasn't going to be free. Time for surgeon number two. This one was even worst. The consultation seemed fine. He seemed like a competent man so I agreed to let him do the surgery. He wanted me to lose weight first so I got started trying my best to do that. I went in for my pre-surgery visit. To his surprise, certainly not to mine, I had only lost 8 pounds. He didn't feel that was enough. My answer to him was "if I was effective at losing weight on my own I wouldn't be getting surgery." He offered to do a different surgery, and then I offered to get my refund and find another surgeon.

FINALLY!! A friend of mine who experienced weight loss success after having surgery referred me to her surgeon. I setup a consultation with him as quickly as possible and was so excited to find a surgeon who was comfortable enough to operate on a 440 pound man. As excited as I was to have potentially found something that would help me become healthier, I was still struggling in faith. What if I come up with all of this out of pocket money, make this drastic change to my body and still end up not losing weight? I was still mentally imprisoned by my past failures. I had to stop playing like an unbothered superhero and allow people who cared to speak encouraging words over me. I found a support group, I let my close family and friends know what I was doing. I was concerned that people would frown on surgery, but I was so desperate for change I didn't even care if anyone approved or disapproved. I was doing this for me! To my surprise, everyone was so excited and supportive.

By everyone, I mean all of those who truly cared. Some of the people I expected to be the most excited seemed quite nonchalant about my endeavors. If we're not careful, we can allow something like that to make us bitter and miss out on all of the wonderful and unexpected people that God has waiting on the sidelines to cheer us on. Not all, but most of my greatest support came from my siblings, social media support groups, co-workers, a few friends, some family and many people I've never met in person. However, I find that the most important encouragement comes from me to me. If I could tear myself down with negative thoughts, surely I could build myself up with the word of God. So no, I'm not a GQ model or athletic sex symbol, but I am *fearfully and wonderfully made.*

Chapter 4

Good Morning Sunshine

I have a friend who texts me first thing in the morning every now and then with the words – "Good morning sunshine". It's extra special because this particular friend does not like texting, but prefers phone calls. I do not like phone calls, but prefer texting. So when I receive this text I smile knowing someone who cares about me is willing to do something unselfish to wish me well. This makes me smile so big because I'm reminded that it's a brand new day. With a new day come new mercies, new opportunities and new chances to be better than I was the day before.

I remember when I was a young boy and I would spend the night at my grandmother's house. The smell of maple smoked bacon and freshly brewed coffee would wake me up early in the morning. I'd turn over in bed and see sunlight radiating through the windows. I'd hear my grandmother in the kitchen singing "Sweet Jesus, sweet Jesus, He's the lily of the valley, bright and morning star". Oh what memories!!! Morning time was pretty sweet in those days, and by the grace of God they are sweet again. My grandmother is no longer here to call me her "MaineyRat" (my sister was "MissyCat"). My mother is no longer here to call me her baby, but if only they could see me now. They were already proud of me while they were living, but they would be absolutely beside themselves with joy right about now. I don't know exactly how Heaven is setup, but I hope God is allowing them to peep down and see the fruits of their labor.

On November 1, 2012 I had a procedure called Duodenal Switch. This surgery is amongst the most invasive and challenging weight loss surgeries that are performed. I was so determined and ready for change that I was up and walking as soon as the nurses allowed me. In pain and all, I was ready to start! I walked and walked and walked around the nurse's station as much as I could. One nurse even tried to stop me and asked me to slow down. Oh no mam!! I've been slow for long enough! It's time to get moving. I was walking marathons around other patients who had much less invasive surgeries. The nurses were so impressed. I was truly ready for change. I had sacrificed too much at this point for this not to work out.

At this point I was preparing myself to dive head first into the challenging work.

Contrary to what some people believe, weight loss surgery is NOT an easy way out. There is still a great deal of effort that must be done by the patient if challenging goals are to be met. Weight loss surgery basically forced my body to cooperate with my efforts. There are many cases where a person gets surgery and don't lose much weight, or regain the weight they lose. It happens, and one of my biggest fears was that I wouldn't lose much at all or end up regaining as in the past. That's why each year I celebrate my "surgiversary". Each year that I'm able to keep the weight off is a huge accomplishment for me.

I started making it easy on myself to stick to a healthier way of eating by making it hard on myself to eat the wrong things. I got rid of all of the bad snacks in my desk and pantry. You can't eat it, if you don't have it. I

like crunchy snacks but chips are not good
when you're trying to lose weight. So I made
sure I had protein rich snacks handy at all
times. Protein chips, low carb trail mix, or nuts.

The greatest challenge has been
incorporating exercise in my daily routine. I'm
a busy hard-working man. On top of that, I
enjoy eating, watching action movies,
shopping and traveling. I honestly do NOT
enjoy exercising. However, I do enjoy the
results of exercise so it must be done. I started
walking early in the mornings before work. I
started walking for 30 minutes, then 45
minutes, then an hour. I was gradually
working my way up. As the pounds began to
come off, I slowly worked my way up to
jogging.

The results have been astonishing. I lost 50 pounds during the first month. I'm going by memory, but I believe I lost my first hundred pounds by week 10. My doctor rejoiced with me as I was able to say goodbye to blood pressure pills and the BiPap machine. I also no longer needed medication to help me deal with Acid Reflux. I could walk for long periods of time without back and knee pain. For the first time in my life, I physically felt like a normal young man. The only downside is how cold I feel in the winters now. But that's nothing a nice coat can't remedy.

Speaking of coats, besides the amazing health improvement – the wardrobe has been so refreshing. I can shop wherever I want! That's something most people take for granted, but it's something I have a special appreciation for. I get so many compliments on my attire now. If you see me now then you'll probably understand why I was very frustrated with the limited selection of clothing that was available for obese men – especially clothes that accommodated my massive and awkward shape. I went from 440 pounds to 190. This only took me a year and a few months to accomplish.

Here's a breakdown of my clothing size comparison.

	Before	After
Shirt	5-6XL	Slim fit Medium
Neck	22	15 ½
Pants	56	33
Coat	62	38 (40 Slim)

The real challenge after losing any amount of weight is maintaining the loss. I already found out the hard way that unrealistic diets do not work. I had to develop a new permanent way of eating that I could adhere to in order to reduce my chance of regain. To lose weight, I stopped eating rice, pasta, bread, fried foods, and sugar. I drunk water and used sugar free add-ins for flavor. Once I reached my goal I was able to re-add some of the foods I enjoy, such as rice, in small portions. This new way of eating is working just fine because I love fish, shrimp, crab, chicken, steak, soups and salads.

You ever heard the phrase "what it takes to get here, it takes to stay here"? Well I found that to be true during this weight loss journey. It takes diligence, will power and discipline. It seems like I'm tested on every hand. The occasional complimentary treats in the office, free bread placed on the table at restaurants, and a busy schedule that makes fast food appealing. On top of that, sometimes I crave something that just isn't healthy. I've learned to be discipline enough to say no. As much as I love a fresh and hot donut, I love being slim more. I let my progress be my motivation to say no when necessary. Just because something is offered doesn't mean it has to be accepted.

Anyone can look at my social media pages and see that I've taken lots of pictures during this journey. The pictures keep me accountable. I don't ever want to look at one of my slim pictures and say, "I certainly miss him". Having so many people look to me for motivation also inspires me to keep maintaining my health. If my success can encourage someone, my failure could possibly discourage someone. That's something I just

don't want on my conscience. This journey is
so much bigger than me and I'm both honored
and in awe about that.

Chapter 5

I'm Not Always a Morning Person

The high praise for my weight loss success has been overwhelming, humbling and honoring. However, I must admit, I'm not always perfect. I didn't reach my goal because I got it right every day. Imperfection is one of the most common discouragers for many of us. We think that since we didn't lose any weight last week, we might as well pig-out at the buffet today. How many dreams and aspirations have we given up on because it didn't work out the first time?

I'm not particularly proud of this but there were days when I ate a cookie while I should've been eating a salad. I lounged on the sofa when I should've been outside running. I even remember standing in line at the Godiva boutique purchasing milk

chocolate and thinking to myself "Don't do it
Abraham!! Get out of the line!! Step away!!"
But I didn't step away. I purchased the
delicious chocolate. I ate a little of it when I
got home and placed the rest on my
nightstand. I kid you not when I say this.
When I woke up the next morning the
chocolate wrappings were empty and there
were chocolate smudges on my face and
fingers. I actually ate the chocolate in my
sleep. Please don't ask me how this is possible,
but it happened. You can take a moment and
laugh now, because I certainly am.

I've learned that it's just too hard to be
perfect and it's unreasonable for us to hold
ourselves hostage to such an unrealistic
standard. This doesn't mean we should stop
trying and pressing. It means we should be
quick to forgive ourselves when we fall short.

It also means that we should empower ourselves to make healthy decisions. How? I wouldn't have eaten those chocolates in my sleep if I hadn't purchased so many in the first place. Since I did purchase them, I should have placed them in the pantry and had a bottle of water on my night stand instead. This way if I just had to reach for something it would be something that wouldn't set me back calorie count wise. Godiva milk chocolate is still my favorite and there's absolutely nothing wrong with me eating them. It's just not good for me to over-eat them. *All things in moderation.* What's good to us is not necessarily good for us.

During my many years of being obese food was my main enjoyment. I was in too much pain to go out and really enjoy life the way I wanted to. I was too embarrassed to be around crowds. So staying home with a good meal, or keeping myself extra busy with work and church were my comforts. If nothing was going on with church or work, then it was food that kept me company. In my journey to better health I had to change this method of comfort to something healthier. Eating now is all about nourishment. Now before you start thinking I'm some health fanatic - I still enjoy good food. I wouldn't dare lie to you and say I only eat lettuce and bean sprouts. I eat what I have a taste for. If it's something that has a lot of calories then I make sure I don't eat very much of it at all, especially if I missed my important morning jog that day.

My mentality about food has changed. I no longer look at it as a comfort mechanism. As far as I'm concerned, food is fuel. If I'm stressed, I need to go for a walk, jog or run. I need to do some push-ups and stomach crunches. Most importantly, I need to pray. Doing these things won't hurt me, but will push me to become the best me I can be. Friends, life is stressful. Things happen outside of our control all of the time. However, this is no excuse to succumb to unhealthy and unfruitful behaviors for comfort. Doing harm to yourself is not going to stop your boss from being a tyrant. Overeating is not going to stop your marriage from being turbulent. Overindulging in alcohol is not going to get your children to obey. Staying up all night and not getting adequate rest is not going to cause your business to become profitable. Taking your frustration out on the faithful few in your ministry is not going to cause the unfaithful many to start cooperating. It's important to us and those around us that we find healthy ways to deal with the inevitable frustrations of life.

Unpleasant situations will present themselves. This is inevitable so let's be prepared.

The nature of my job is dealing with tight deadlines, multitasking, organizing events and dealing with people for eight plus hours a day. In a job of this nature it is ridiculous to expect every day to be smooth and stress free. It's just not going to happen. There are days when I need to be a miracle worker. There are days when I need to answer to my superior within an hour but the people with the answer can't get with me until the next day. I have to be prepared to deal with stress and annoyances. Does this sound familiar? Your life may be different than mine but we all face these types of challenges. I find that equipping my physical self enables me to handle my day with poise, peace and joy.

First, I start my day with prayer. Prayer is not

optional for me, it's mandatory. Secondly, I exercise. I go for a morning jog because I find that it's most effective in helping me maintain my weight loss. Thirdly, I say no to unhealthy breakfast. As much as I'd love a fresh hot donut, sausage and cheese kolache or cream-filled stuffed pastry - I say no! I could probably enjoy a little of this without gaining weight but eating something that will trigger my cravings for high calorie foods just isn't a good start to my day.

It's important to discover what works for you. An early morning jog may not be possible for you due to your schedule. Perhaps an evening gym session would work better. I eat peanuts for a crunchy snack, but you may be allergic to peanuts. Perhaps celery and carrots would be a better alternative. I had surgery to lose weight quickly due to my health problems and also to force my body to cooperate with my efforts. Surgery may not be the best option for you. You may not be overweight enough, or maybe the expense is just too great for you right now. Perhaps seeking advice from your doctor, nutritionist and fitness instructor would be a much better start for you. We may have to use different methods due to our different circumstances, but the goal is similar. We all want to live our best life possible.

The key to weight loss success for me has not been perfection. The key has been to not give up – EVER! Wake up every morning forgiving everyone and yourself for anything that happened that shouldn't have happened. Forgive everyone and yourself for anything that should've happened but didn't. Every day you wake up is another chance. If we hold ourselves hostage to what we didn't accomplish before, we'll never see victory. It's time to move forward.

This is good news for you. Perhaps your goal is a better career, to get married, have children, ministry work, obtain a degree or start your own business. Whatever your goal is, just like me - you don't have to be perfect to reach it.

"Death and life are in the power of the tongue: and they that love it shall eat the fruit thereof." {Proverbs 18:21}

I have countless messages from people saying "I just can't lose the weight". Sometimes I hear people saying things like "I just can't get this business off the ground". "I just can't deal with these kids anymore". "I'm sick of this marriage". The first thing that must be done is to stop declaring what you're not willing to live with. It's not that you can't, you just haven't yet. You haven't tapped in to what your body will respond to yet. You haven't quite made the right business connections yet. You haven't found the most effective discipline techniques for your children yet. You haven't discovered the root issue that is disturbing the peace of your marriage yet. I too hindered myself with the "I can't" attitude. When I wised up, I was able to break out of that rut and declare "I can" until finally "I did".

So many people have asked me what my secret is. I don't have a secret but my advice is this - pray for guidance, research for methods and follow instructions. Guidance will lead you to the correct resources and place you in the company of those who have made it where you are trying to go. Researching optional methods will open your mind to new ideas that may be different and scary, but ultimately effective. Following instructions is absolutely essential to the success of accomplishing any task. I've had people to ask me what I did to lose weight. I share the story with them but they do something totally different and of course don't get the results they were hoping for.

I'm feeling better and looking better. I'm happier and healthier. However, the greatest joy I've received from this journey is to know that many people are being inspired by it. I never dreamed that people would look at me and be inspired to be healthier, or to fight a little harder to fulfil their dreams. Being able to enjoy life is phenomenal. The ability to

dress the way I've always wanted to is great.
Enjoying a meal without being fearful of
gaining weight is refreshing. To feel normal
while enjoying the company of family and
friends is priceless. Motivating and inspiring
people to trust God to empower them for a
better life – that's the glory! My life has
changed for the better. When I compare where
I was just a few years ago to where I am now –
it is truly like night and day.

Thank you for reading. The journey
continues....

www.ingramcontent.com/pod-product-compliance
Lightning Source LLC
Chambersburg PA
CBHW071116280526
45787CB00003B/1073